The Basics  Vegan Lifestyle

How to Live Meat-Free and Dairy-Free

By Lewis Haas
©2015

The Basics of a Healthy Vegan Lifestyle:
How to Live Meat-Free and Dairy-Free
All rights reserved
May 28, 2015
Copyright ©2015 One Jacked Monkey, LLC
onejackedmonkey.com
ISBN-13: 978-1514131596
ISBN-10: 1514131595

No part of this book may be reproduced or transmitted in any form or by any means, electronic or mechanical, including photocopying, recording or by any information storage and retrieval system, without the permission in writing from One Jacked Monkey, LLC.

Disclaimer

Although the author and publisher have made every effort to ensure that the information in this book was correct at press time, the author and publisher do not assume and hereby disclaim any liability to any party for any loss, damage, or disruption caused by errors or omissions, whether such errors or omissions result from negligence, accident, or any other cause.

This is an informational guide and is not intended as a substitute for medical or professional services. Readers are urged to consult a variety of sources such as their medical doctor, dietitian or nutritionist. The information expressed herein is the opinion of the author and is not intended to reflect upon any particular person or company. The author shall have no responsibility or liability with respect to any loss or damage caused, or alleged, by the information or application contained in this guide. One Jacked Monkey, LLC, and the author are not associated nor represent any product or vendor mentioned in this book.

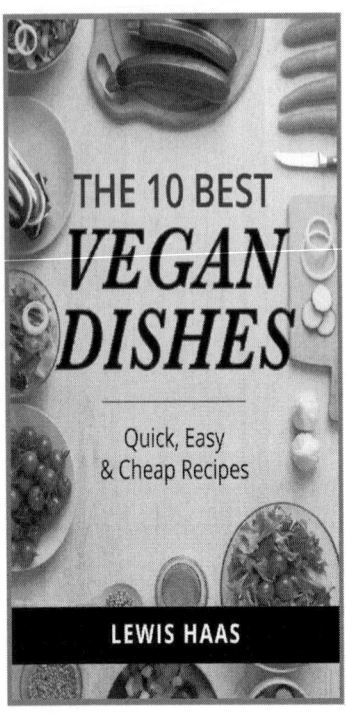

Grab the
10 Best
Vegan Recipes
That Are Cheap, Quick and Easy to Make...FREE!

"The 10 Best Vegan Dishes" has just what you need to satisfy your appetite, to spare your money and to save you time:

- 3 Awesome Varieties of Breakfast
- 4 Different Delicious Lunches
- 3 Distinct Dinner Dishes
- Many tips and notes to get the most out of every dish
- Options and alternatives for some recipes

Have you struggled with finding GOOD vegan recipes that are easy to make? Are you needing to find recipes that are tasty AND cheap?

With 10 vegan recipes and a number of options and alternatives to some of the dishes, you will have plenty of vibrant, flavorful meals that will fill you up, keep you healthy and looking forward to your next meal.

Get this book FREE

Go to http://eepurl.com/bfE46z to get a free copy sent to your email

Table of Contents

Introduction 1
Chapter 1: Flexitarian, Pescatarian, Vegetarian, Vegan, Confuse-itarian? 7
Chapter 2: Why Be Vegan? 15
Chapter 3: Vegan Nutrition 23
    Protein 24
    Vitamin B_{12} 26
    Vitamin D & Calcium 27
        Vitamin D 27
        Calcium 28
Chapter 4: Now That You Are Committed 31
Chapter 5: 5 Day Sample Meal Plan 41
Chapter 6: One Size Never Fits All 59
Chapter 7: Eating Out 65
Chapter 8: Types of Vegans 69
Thank You 72
About the Author 73
References 74
Citations 82

Introduction

Have you ever wondered why New Year's Resolutions never seem to stick? On January 1st, people are determined to fulfill the promise they made to themselves. Yet, January flies by without their intended outcome. Due to professional and personal commitments, their goal only gets half completed. Many people give up or feel guilty for being unable to stick to their goals. If you're one of those people, stop blaming yourself. Lifestyle habits are hard to break, or even impossible, if there isn't some guidance or a plan to put in place. You may have an admirable goal and your inability to meet it has nothing to do with your conviction. All you need is a little support and guidance along the way. You need a concrete plan to fulfill your goal.

This handbook is the support and the guidance new vegans need to make a lasting lifestyle change. New vegans come from many different backgrounds and have diverse reasons for committing to this lifestyle. This book examines veganism from a number of perspectives and emphasizes flexible adaptation to the ideas put forth in the text.

One of the book's main themes is that veganism is a return to the more natural, intuitive way of eating. The Standard American Diet (SAD) is mainly comprised of an exorbitant amount of animal products and food from boxes, only made edible by adding chemicals, sugars, fats and extra sodium to them. Veganism, however, is a more natural way of eating and dates back to our hunter-gatherer way of life. Humans should naturally eat a diet mainly composed of fruits, tender greens and vegetables, seeds, nuts and legumes. Meat was a luxury to have once in a while. It certainly was not the staple of every meal.

The first chapter provides an overview of the different types of diets that limit the consumption of animal products. The chapter proceeds to explain the important ethical, environmental, and health distinctions between veganism and vegetarianism in order to make the claim that veganism is a better choice than other diets that only limit the consumption of animal products. The second chapter flows into a detailed discussion about the ethical, health and environmental reasons to become a vegan.

The third chapter is the benefits of vegan nutrition and to dispel any myths related to veganism. While the moral and the environmental reasons for veganism receive little to no contention, many non-vegans question the vegan's ability to meet complete nutritional requirements. Furthermore, I'll cover concerns of nutritional deficiencies in veganism. The book looks at the role of protein, vitamin D, vitamin B_{12} and calcium in the vegan diet.

Chapter four helps new vegans discern what foods to buy and what items should always be in the pantry or fridge. This is to ensure a tasty and affordable vegan meal is never inconvenient. The chapter also discusses how to make your vegan lifestyle affordable by providing suggestions about where to buy food and the types of foods that should be considered staples. (Hint: fresh, seasonal produce!)

The fifth chapter displays how the aforementioned foods can be used to create delicious, vegan meals. The fifth chapter includes a five-day 2,000 calories sample meal plan. Each day includes breakfast, lunch, dinner and at least two snacks. The meal plans are general suggestions, can be adapted to suit your needs or simply used as inspiration for your own meal plans. The emphasis is on meeting personal preferences *and* nutritional requirements.

The sixth and seventh chapters discuss the effects your new vegan lifestyle may have on other aspects of your life. The sixth chapter focuses on animal products used in textile and cosmetic industries. Ultimately, the choice to expand your veganism to textile and cosmetic industries is up to you. New vegans may want to do this gradually. The seventh chapter offers tips for eating out with non-vegans.

Chapter eight delves into the different types of veganism and suggests that beginners to veganism focus more on making veganism work for them, rather than focusing on how to fit into a subset vegan lifestyle.

Lastly, I want you to know that veganism is a lifestyle change dedicated to greater love and respect for all beings on this planet. Whenever snares or roadblocks appear, new vegans should take solace in their kinder, gentler, and more peaceful way of living. With a plan and noble causes, new vegans following this book will stick to their resolutions and convictions for years to come.

Lewis Haas

Chapter 1: Flexitarian, Pescatarian, Vegetarian, Vegan, Confuse-itarian?

Most everyone likes labels since they simplify complex and nuanced ideas that are otherwise difficult to discern. However, everyone also likes to be thought of as individual, which creates the paradox of creating so many terms that labels become pointless. In fact, some people label themselves "label-free" which perfectly encapsulates this labeling madness.

Perhaps nowhere in our modern society does this labeling paradox appear than in the numerous terms for dietary lifestyles. These lifestyles include:
- Vegan
- Raw Vegan
- Lacto-Ovo Vegetarian
- Pescatarian
- Flexitarian
- Paleo
- Macrobiotic

The list goes on and on.

This introductory chapter will first clear up the differences between diets that restrict the consumption of animal products. It will then explain why veganism (whether you choose to be raw vegan, raw till 4 vegan, etc.) is by far the best and easiest-to-follow dietary lifestyle.

The term "flexitarian" combines *flexible* with *vegetarian,* exactly as its terminology implies. Followers cut back on their meat and seafood consumption, but do not eliminate it. There is not a set amount of meat or seafood you are allowed to eat, but the general consensus is that followers still follow a predominately plant-based diet and are completely meatless at least once a week.[1] There are no rules as to what type of meat or seafood is consumed. Dairy and egg products are permitted in this diet.

Pescatarians are stricter flexitarians since they refrain from meat (poultry, pork, beef) but eat fish. This term combines the Italian word for fish, *pesce* and *vegetarian*.[2] Some pescatarians consider themselves vegetarian, but they are simply a more restrictive version of a flexitarian. Like flexitarians, pescatarians often choose to limit their consumption of animal products for health reasons. Like flexitarians, there is no limit to their dairy and egg consumption. Pescatarianism and flexitarianism are among the most common dietary lifestyles that are based on the reduction or limitation of animal products. A study conducted by The Vegetarian Resource Group discovered roughly 30-40% of the U.S. population is at least interested in choosing to order or cook meals without meat.[3]

Flexitarians and pescatarians are not true vegetarians as they still consume meat. True vegetarians never eat fish, poultry, or shellfish. Many vegetarians eat dairy and eggs and some will refrain from eating foods that possibly contain animal products, such as chicken stock and gelatin.[4] Vegetarians who choose to eat dairy products, but not eggs, are called lacto-vegetarians. Vegetarians who eat egg, but not dairy products, are called ovo-vegetarians. Finally, the most common type of vegetarian is a lacto-ovo vegetarian. These vegetarians consume dairy and egg products but restrict all other animal products.

The Vegan Society defines veganism as a lifestyle that avoids food or other products whose production or distribution resulted in the harm, suffering, and exploitation of animals.[5] In layman's terms this means that authentic vegans eat no meat, poultry, fish, shellfish, dairy, eggs, and other animal products such as honey and gelatin. Some vegans also choose to refrain from buying or using any non-edible products made from animals such as leather and wool.

These are the main dietary lifestyles that revolve around restricting the consumption of animal products. Readers new to these lifestyles may wonder why people choose to be vegan rather than these other options, particularly vegetarianism. Many vegetarians believe that by not eating meat they are staying ethical and healthy. However, this is not the case due to the cruelty of the dairy industry and the fact that Western Vegetarian diets tend to be no more healthful in many respects than standard meat-eating diets.

Vegans see the dairy industry as one of the most barbaric parts of the animal industry. In many ways, the dairy industry is in fact crueler than the meat industry because animals survive longer under more torturous conditions. For example, due to the use of Bovine Growth Hormones, most female dairy cows are forced to

The Basics of a Healthy Vegan Lifestyle

produce more than ten times the natural amount of milk to feed humans.[6] This causes their udders to swell to the point where they can hardly walk. Likewise, most dairy cows are killed after just four or five years even though a cow's natural lifespan should exceed two decades. Their short lives are spent in captivity, never to see the outdoors.[7] Their bodies are pushed to the point of total destruction. Male calves, or baby cows, are taken from their mothers almost immediately and are slaughtered in just a few months. To continuously produce milk, female cows are repeatedly impregnated which puts a considerable strain on their bodies.[8]

Egg-laying hens and their babies are among the most tortured animals sold for human consumption. Baby male chicks are slaughtered immediately after birth since they have little value on the market. The vast majority of egg-laying hens are kept in battery cages which are windowless cages crammed so much that each chicken doesn't even have space the size of a sheet of paper to themselves.[9] The term cage-free is used in the livestock industry to soothe concerned consumers who learn about the battery cage system. However, cage-free hens have slightly more space than battery cage hens. The tragic, unnatural conditions hens live in cause them to attack one another in desperation. Therefore, many farmers will actually remove a part of the hens' beaks, which leads to chronic, permanent pain.[10] Thus, vegetarians are just as guilty as meat-eaters when it comes to supporting the continued suffering of animals.

One of the other main reasons people turn to vegetarianism is to reap the health benefits. Many vegetarians increase their dairy consumption to substitute for the meat they no longer eat. However, dairy is not a health food by any stretch. In fact, recent studies have come out seriously questioning dairy's health benefits. We were taught to believe that the high levels of calcium in dairy promote strong bones and prevent osteoporosis. In reality, countries with some of the lowest rates of dairy consumption have low rates of osteoporosis. Dairy also appears to have no impact on preventing broken bones. In fact, it tends to do more harm than good. It contributes to additional health problems like indigestion and heart disease due to the high levels of fat.[11] Even scarier, numerous studies have linked dairy consumption to higher risks of certain types of cancers such as prostate, testicular, ovarian and breast cancers.[12]

Thus the most substantial dietary difference between veganism and vegetarianism is the consumption of dairy products. The consumption of these dairy products are neither ethically sound nor beneficial to ones overall health, yet these are some of the main reasons people choose to be vegetarians. Veganism, therefore, is the only dietary lifestyle that successfully leads its people to become more ethical and healthy human beings. Throw the rest of the labels away. Simple, matter-of-fact veganism is the solution.

Lewis Haas

Chapter 2: Why Be Vegan?

Every vegan out there can tell you about the gamut of reactions they've received from friends and even total strangers when they declare they are vegan. People react with bafflement, respect, confusion, amusement, and even concern about a vegan's nutritional well-being. Regardless of their response, people almost always ask, "Why?" Luckily for you new vegans out there, this is a very easy question to answer. Health, environmental, and ethical reasons make adapting to a vegan lifestyle the easiest choice you can make. In fact, the harder question to answer is, "Why not?"

The exorbitant amount of meat in the Standard American Diet (SAD) has very little in common with mankind's natural hunter-gatherer state. Dr. Douglas Graham, a renowned raw vegan medical professional, athlete, and author of numerous books on vegan lifestyles gracefully explains mankind's natural diet.[13] For thousands of years, mankind relied on a diet comprised of fruits and tender greens, with little grain (until the evolution of cereal agriculture), some nuts, legumes and seeds, and limited meat consumption from hunted game. In essence, humans are what Dr. Graham calls "frugivores" or beings that eat mainly fruit with some tender, green vegetables.[14] True, this diet was not vegan, but it does attest to man's natural plant-based lifestyle.

There is evidence to suggest the idea of veganism dates back to the Greco-Roman Empire. For instance, the Greek philosopher Porphory's argues in his work, *On Abstinence from Animal Food,* that killing animals is unjust. He argues that if a person thinks hurting animals is inhumane then that person should not eat meat or use any other products derived from animal suffering.[15]

The dawn of modern day vegetarians and vegans occurred in the early 19th century with proponents such as Dr. William Lambe and the poet Percy Bysshe Shelley, who wrote works such as *A Vindication of a Natural Diet.* Donald Watson came up with the term vegan in 1944 with a joint commission of other non-dairy vegetarians. They chose the term vegan because it took the beginning and end of the word vegetarian.[16]

Results from a 2013 study estimates that over 7 million Americans identify themselves as vegan, which is double the vegan population from 2009![17] The number of American vegans has doubled in the past five years due to the amazing health benefits, eco-friendly way of living and moral righteousness vegans experience.

The most immediate and personal effects of abstaining from animal products are the health benefits. The renowned epidemiologist, Dr. Colin Campbell, undertook a massive study that compared rates of diseases in the United States to rates of disease in rural China. The United States has a high-fat, animal, and processed food-based diet. Rural Chinese follow mainly vegan, plant-based diets. The results of Dr. Campbell's study were shocking. Years of research indicated there was a significant correlation between eating animal products and the diseases that afflict many Americans. Diseases now known to be caused in part by the Standard American Diet include: cancer, heart disease, diabetes, various auto-immune diseases, obesity, and diseases of the bones, eyes, kidneys, and brain. Essentially, meat and high-fat processed food destroys the human body. Where incidents of heart disease and diabetes run rampant in the United Sates, they are almost non-existent in vegan societies.[18]

What exactly is it about the vegan diet that makes its followers some of the healthiest people on the planet? The vegan diet is full of vitamins, minerals, proteins, and healthful fats and carbohydrates that the human body is evolutionarily designed to consume. To cite Winston J. Craig's helpful summary:

> *Vegan diets are usually higher in dietary fiber, magnesium, folic acid, vitamin C and E, iron, and phytochemicals, and they tend to be lower in calories, saturated fat and cholesterol....a vegan diet appears to be useful for increasing the intake of protective nutrients and phytochemicals and for minimizing the intake of dietary factors implicated in several chronic disease.* (Craig, 2009 March 11, p. 1627S).[19]

The Basics of a Healthy Vegan Lifestyle

The inhumane slaughter of animals for their meat and other body parts has turned many peoples' stomachs and minds towards veganism. There are a number of ethical reasons to go vegan. First of all, humankind could not survive if everyone were to adopt Western diets, which often includes eating an animal product or two at every meal. The strain on natural, limited resources in order to eat animal products is frankly downright selfish. It takes up to ten pounds of grain to produce just one pound of meat.[20]

The meat industry tries to sell the public an idyllic, guilt-free version of animal production where animals are kept in open pastures with their offspring. According to them, animals die a natural, painless death and are then sold as meat. What they portray is furthest from the truth. Instead, most animals live out short, desolate lives in Concentrated Animal Feeding Operations (CAFO), commonly referred to as Factory Farms. Cows, chickens, pigs and turkeys are the most common species found living in these dire conditions. These animals live in almost complete darkness, receive little to no veterinary care, are forcibly and repeatedly impregnated and have shortened lives due to premature slaughter and disease. They live in unsanitary, polluted conditions with little space of their own. They are given ample amounts of medication just to keep them alive in these conditions.[21]

Dairy cows are killed at 3-4 years of age, though they naturally live more than two decades. Each year hundreds of millions of male chickens are killed as soon as they are born.[22] There are no guidelines in place to protect fish from cruelty so many fish are cut open and have their organs ripped out while still conscious.[23] Factory-farmed fish have some of the bleakest lives. Conditions are often so barbaric that half of all fish die before they are ready to be slaughtered for consumption. The encasements that hold the fish are dirty and full of bacteria and parasites. Fish routinely starve to death.[24]

Vegans who choose to not buy or wear animal products, such as wool, further abide by ethical guidelines. Sheep are routinely wounded in the shearing process because employees are paid by the amount of wool they gather rather than by the hour. During the sheering process, large amounts of skin is accidentally removed from the sheep. And, baby sheep routinely die due to extreme conditions and starvation.[25]

Many people are turning towards a vegan lifestyle due to the animal production industry's harmful effects on the environment. It wastes resources, contributes to pollution and has horrible public health ramifications. One third of the world's water supply is used for animal production, which includes meat and dairy products.[26] Livestock production drains resources that could be used to feed people. For instance, over a billion tons of grains are fed to animals each year.[27] Livestock also contributes to significant deforestation and greenhouse gas emissions. Animal grazing actually takes up 25% of earth's land. As the earth becomes more populated, land is destroyed to make room for animals. Likewise, animals actually produce more greenhouse gas than the much more commonly cited transportation culprit.[28]

Finally, factory farming is a huge contributor to antibiotic resistance and superbugs worldwide. Over 80% of all antibiotics used in the United States are given to livestock rather than to humans. These livestock, as The National Resources Defense Council explains, are not sick.

Instead, these antibiotics are used to keep bacteria from growing out of hand in the squalor conditions that CAFOs force animals to live in. Eventually bacteria becomes resistant to antibiotics, which creates superbugs and strains of disease that becomes more and more difficult to treat.[29]

It is often asked, "Why vegan?" But, the real tricky question they should ask now is, "Why not vegan?"

Chapter 3: Vegan Nutrition

The World Health Organization's (W.H.O.) guidelines for a healthy diet indicate a vegan-like lifestyle.[30] They urge that less than 10% of your total calories should come from freestanding sugars found in processed foods and desserts. They also recommend a low-fat diet in which less than 30% of your calories should come from fat. The W.H.O. strongly urges these fats should be from plant or nut sources rather than from animal products. Finally, salt intake should be limited.[31] In essence, the best diet as recommended by the world's premier health authority, is the vegan diet.

Despite recommendations by the W.H.O., many Americans are wary of following a vegan diet due to the myth that this lifestyle creates nutritional deficiencies. The most commonly cited deficiencies associated with a vegan diet include a lack of protein, vitamin B_{12}, vitamin D and calcium. These concerns are often unwarranted and there are ways to ensure as a vegan, you meet these dietary needs.

Protein

The livestock industry has done an excellent job of convincing consumers that protein can only be sufficiently found in meat and other animal products. There are several problems with this claim. The first is that the United States Department of Agriculture (USDA) grossly overstates how much protein is actually needed. The second is that more nutritionally dense protein is actually found in plants rather than in animals. In fact, animal protein is harmful, especially in the quantities that most Americans consume them. The current U.S. government nutrition guidelines suggest Americans receive a minimum of 10% to a maximum of 35% of their calories from protein.[32] These ranges, particularly the 35% suggestion, are ludicrous. The average American consumes nowhere near this 35% mark. In fact, kinesiologists don't even suggest this amount for bodybuilders and premier athletes! Instead, they recommend around 25%.[33] In fact, protein levels as high as 20% have been known to have adverse effects. Thomas Campbell, author of *The China Study* cites a monumental study that found mice fed a high-protein diet had much higher rates of liver cancer than mice fed a low-protein diet (around 5%).[34] Moreover, the minimum 10% is actually far more protein than the human body actually needs. In reality, humans only need about 5-6% of their daily calories from protein. The 10% recommended is a safety net.[35]

It is still entirely possible for vegans to have a high-level protein diet. Here are a few examples:

- One cup of cooked lentils = ~20 grams of protein
- A small serving of tofu = ~12 grams of protein
- Two slices of whole wheat bread = ~10 grams of protein
- Two tablespoons of peanut butter = ~8 grams

Green vegetables like spinach, kale, broccoli and Brussels sprouts are packed with protein for their low-caloric value. Truthfully, most food contains protein. For example, a serving of blackberries contains 2 grams of protein. Finally, to reach the USDA recommendations for minimum protein, a person eating 2,000 calories needs 50 grams, or 200 calories, of protein per day. As a good example, two pieces of toast with two tablespoons of peanut butter and a simple serving of tofu curry with vegetables would bring you close to your daily protein goal.

Vitamin B_{12}

Vitamin B_{12} is an essential vitamin for healthy red blood cells, for preventing anemia (lack of red blood cells) and for the body's construction of DNA.[36] It is one of the main arguments against veganism because many people believe B_{12} is only found in animal products. While B_{12} is naturally found in animal products, there are ways for vegans to obtain proper amounts of B_{12}.[37] Some vegans choose to get their B_{12} through supplements. For example, many cereals are fortified with B_{12}. Vegans can also take a daily B_{12} supplement. However, there are natural ways to get B_{12} as well. For instance, nutritional yeast is a delicious, vegan super food. Two tablespoons of nutritional yeast provide nearly half of your daily B_{12} needs. Some vegans choose not to use vitamin B_{12} supplements since some are processed from animal intestines.[38] However, because B_{12} deficiencies cause all sorts of horrible side effects, vegans starting out may want to consider supplementation. Consult your vegan-friendly physician for what is appropriate for you.

Vitamin D & Calcium

Some people believe Vitamin D and Calcium are only found in dairy and meat products. Many people decide to forgo veganism and to a lesser extent, vegetarianism, because they fear these nutritional deficiencies. On the contrary, veganism is perfectly adequate to meet these nutritional requirements with careful selection and recommendations by a qualified health care professional.

Vitamin D

Vitamin D is important for bone health. Vitamin D is naturally found in very limited food sources, namely fatty fish, egg yolks, and to a smaller extent, cheese and beef. The majority of the U.S. population gets Vitamin D from fortified milk, breakfast cereals, non-dairy milks, and orange juice. What most people don't realize is that we get most of our Vitamin D from the sun.[39] The amount of time spent in the sun depends on how dark your skin is. Fair skinned people may need only ten minutes while olive skinned people need twenty minutes. Those with the darkest skin tones need closer to one hour of sun.[40] It is best to expose your arms and legs to the sun when seeking to gain Vitamin D from sun exposure. Consult your physician for what is the best fit for you.

Calcium

The dairy industry has been successfully convincing the public for years that milk and dairy are excellent calcium sources necessary to promote strong bones.[41] In reality, milk is quite harmful. Dr. Campbell, author of *The China Study* analyzed his studies and others to demonstrate dairy consumption increased ones' risk of osteoporosis, prostate cancer and numerous autoimmune diseases.[42] Moreover, plant-based calcium is readily available and overall a much better source of this nutrient. Adults should get around 1,000 mg of calcium each day. Calcium can be found in high quantities

The Basics of a Healthy Vegan Lifestyle

in vegetables such as collard greens (266 mg per cup), kale (94 mg per cup), butternut squash (84 mg per cup), and broccoli (62 mg per cup). Plant protein sources also contain calcium such as tofu (250 mg per ½ cup) and garbanzo beans (80 mg per cup). Fruits like figs (10 figs = ~140 mg) and oranges (~60 mg) also contain calcium. As you can see, it is incredibly easy to get your dietary requirements from a vegan diet.

Lewis Haas

Chapter 4: Now That You Are Committed

Congratulations! You've made it this far. You've committed to the vegan lifestyle and are ready to toss out your cancer-causing cheeses and tortured meats. Yet, you've run into one small problem - besides kale and bananas, you may have no idea what you're supposed to be eating! Never fear, this next chapter will explain vegan essentials, where to buy them and how to make a vegan lifestyle affordable for you and your family. Of course, the most important thing to consider when purchasing any food items is whether or not you're actually going to eat it. Sure, kale is a super food, chock full of calcium and protein but if you hate kale—don't buy it! The vegan lifestyle is not restrictive and can adapt to any number of picky eaters or sensitive taste buds.

Below you will find the items I almost always have in my fridge, freezer (though I always prefer fresh over frozen), and cupboard.

Grains & Starches

- oats
- any assortment of the following: brown rice, quinoa, farro, barley, whole-grain or gluten-free pasta, spelt, couscous and any other whole grain you enjoy
- whole-wheat bread. My favorite brand is Ezekiel Bread 4:9 Company. Their flaxseed and cinnamon raisin varieties are my favorites
- some whole-grain or gluten-free flour for baking
- sweet potatoes or yams

Legumes

I always have a few cans for convenience or bulk dry beans to prepare for later. Feel free to mix it up!
- black beans
- dark red kidney beans
- garbanzo beans, also known as, chick peas
- pinto beans
- dried lentils

Nuts & Seeds
- flaxseed
- chia seeds

The Basics of a Healthy Vegan Lifestyle

- almonds, pistachios, walnuts (mix it up!)
- peanut or almond butter

<u>Lots of Vegetables</u>

I try to buy seasonal and local whenever possible, but these are staples no matter the time of year

- spinach, kale or other dark green leafy vegetables
- avocado
- tomatoes
- broccoli
- bell peppers
- cucumber
- zucchini
- baby carrots
- mushrooms

<u>Non-Dairy Alternatives</u>

- almond, soy or rice milk (I always have at least two cartons at home)
- coconut yogurt or soy yogurt (Getting the plain flavor is best since refined sugar or sweeteners are added to the flavored varieties. Add fruit for flavor, instead.)

Fruits
- bananas (I go through two bunches per week)
- apples
- berries
- some sort of tropical fruit whether that be oranges, mango, papaya, etc. (high in vitamin C)
- dates or figs

Spices and Oils
(Use oils sparingly. One serving or less per day)
- olive oil
- coconut oil (olive oil makes sweet baked items taste a bit odd, so I prefer coconut oil)
- salt
- pepper
- cumin
- turmeric
- cilantro
- basil
- curry powder
- garlic
- onions
- chili powder

The Basics of a Healthy Vegan Lifestyle

- cinnamon
- vanilla
- nutmeg
- shredded coconut
- unsweetened cocoa
- nutritional yeast (has a nutty-cheese flavor and is good for you)

<u>Other Protein Sources</u>
- tofu or tempeh (fermented tofu)
- vegan protein powder
- frozen veggie burgers in case of emergency

And there you have it! These are staple items of a vegan diet. I cannot stress enough how important it is to follow your own taste buds though. You won't stick to a diet you don't like it.

The main takeaways here are:
- The bulk of your food should be fresh produce
- Use more spices for flavor
- Use oil sparingly
- A vegan diet is very affordable. The most expensive item on this list is probably $20

USD and that is about a month of vegan protein powder. Most items cost no more than a few bucks.

Some people think vegan and vegetarian diets are expensive because they believe vegan food is only available at pricey health food stores. True, if you buy pricey faux-meats and frozen vegan products at high end grocery stores, then it is possible to spend quite a bit of money on this lifestyle. Overall veganism costs what you are willing to pay and there are number of ways to make it the most affordable lifestyle option out there.

First, the vast majority of the items mentioned above are found at your every day grocery store or farmer's market. Most of the shopping can done at traditional grocery stores and some groceries can be bought at the farmer's markets. Whenever possible, purchase organic and non-GMO foods. Most grocery stores recognize the market for these items and offer them at competitive costs.

It is always preferable to purchase organic products, but the agricultural sector continues to grow many types of produce in a way in which

The Basics of a Healthy Vegan Lifestyle

the difference between organic and non-organic is negligible. These types of produce are called the "The Clean 15." The Clean 15 are:[43]

- onions
- avocado
- sweet corn
- pineapples
- mango
- sweet peas
- asparagus
- kiwi
- cabbage
- eggplant
- cantaloupe
- watermelon
- grapefruit
- sweet potatoes
- sweet onions

Granted, if you save money on these you should always purchase organic from the Dirty Dozen, twelve different produce items that are safest when bought completely organic (produce grown pesticide-free and chemical-free). The Dirty Dozen include:[44]

- peaches
- strawberries

- apples
- blueberries
- nectarines
- bell peppers
- dark green leafy vegetables
- cherries
- potatoes
- grapes
- lettuce

Another way to save money is to buy local whenever possible. Farmer's markets and food co-ops offer competitive prices for their produce. Since these locations tend to be locally owned businesses, many vendors and co-op organizations provide buyers with discounts if they buy in bulk or pledge to buy a certain amount of food every year. Definitely look into these options at the nearest market or food co-op near you.

To conclude, you can buy the $9.00 kale chips or the $12 jar of raw sunflower seed butter, but you could just as easily buy a $2.00 jumbo bag of organic kale and a $3 jar of no-sugar added, natural peanut butter. You could buy a $5.00 smoothie drink, or you could make one of your own at home with produce at a fifth of the

The Basics of a Healthy Vegan Lifestyle

cost. You could buy a $5 box of four veggie burgers or you could buy three cans of beans for $0.50 a can, add some flour and make your own burgers. As you can see, like any other diet, veganism can be as expensive or as cheap as you want to make it.

Lewis Haas

Chapter 5: 5 Day Sample Meal Plan

The following is a five-day sample meal plan for new vegans. This is a 2000 calorie diet, which may be too little or, very unlikely, too much for your dietary needs. However, this should a good base to start from.

Each meal includes ingredients, measurements, and approximated calorie contents. Some offer complete recipes with instructions if the meal is not self-explanatory.

Day 1 (5 Day Sample Meal Plan)
<u>Breakfast: Pumpkin Pie, Protein Packed Oatmeal</u>
- ½ Cup of Canned, Unsweetened Pumpkin
- ½ cup of Dried Oatmeal (Plain)
- 1 tsp. nutmeg
- 1 tsp. cinnamon
- 1 tbsp. brown sugar
- 1 Scoop Vegan Protein Powder
- Water or Non-Dairy Milk

(250 Calories)

<u>Snack: 2 Navel Oranges</u>
(150 Calories)

<u>Lunch: Thai Tofu Coconut Curry w/ Rice (4 Servings)</u>
- Coconut or Olive Oil
- Ginger
- 1 TBSP Curry Powder
- 1 Can Light Coconut Milk
- 2 Heads Bok Choy
- 1 Cup Vegetable Stock
- Chili Powder, to taste
- 2-3 carrots
- 2-3 tomatoes

The Basics of a Healthy Vegan Lifestyle

- One block Extra-Firm Tofu
- 1 cup quinoa
- Lemongrass
- 1 Diced Onion
- 2-3 Garlic Cloves, to taste.

(450 Calories per serving)

Snack: Oil-Free Granola

(Cook in oven at 320 Fahrenheit for 25 minutes stirring every 10)

- 2 cups oats
- 1 cup chopped almonds
- 1 cup chopped dates
- ½ cup pumpkin seeds
- ¼ cup flaxseeds
- 1 tbsp. ground cinnamon
- 1 tbsp. nutmeg
- 2/3 cup maple syrup
- add dried fruit after baking

Inspired by:
(http://simpleveganblog.com/oil-free-granola/)

(1/2 cup is 200 calories)

<u>Dinner: Quinoa Spring Rolls with Red Cabbage, Carrots, Cucumbers and Spinach with sauce of choice</u>

(Cook Quinoa in 2 cups of water for 15-20 minutes

Bake Tofu for 30 or so minute minutes at 400 Fahrenheit)

- one pack of seaweed or Paper Spring Roll Wrappers
- 3/4 cup dried quinoa or brown rice
- 3/4 cup cabbage
- 2 carrots
- 1 cup chopped spinach
- 2 cucumbers
- 1 block extra firm tofu
- Sauce of choice

(Roughly 100 calories in each with sauce. 4 is a suggested serving size)

<u>Desert: Coconut Yogurt with Sweet Bing Cherries</u>
- 8 oz. coconut yogurt, unsweetened
- 1 cup bing cherries

(300 calories)
TOTAL CALORIES = 1800

Day 2 (5 Day Sample Meal Plan)

Breakfast: Chocolate, Banana & Strawberry "Nice Cream" topped with chia seeds and unsweetened, shredded coconuts

- 4 frozen Bananas
- 1.5 cups Strawberries
- 1 tbsp. unsweetened cocoa
- 1 tbsp. agave syrup to taste
- 2 tsp. chia seeds
- 1 tsp. coconut (unsweetened)

(Roughly 600 Calories)

Snack: Avocado Mash on Toast

- 1 tsp. coconut (unsweetened)
- ½ avocado
- 2 pieces of toast
- Salt
- Lemon Juice
- Cilantro

(250 calories)

Lunch: Chickpea Salad (Ground chickpeas and Veganaise) Sandwich with sprouts and Roma tomatoes

Ground Chickpea Salad

The Basics of a Healthy Vegan Lifestyle

(Blend in Food Processor, makes 2 servings)
- 1 can of chickpeas
- 1.5 tbsp. Veganaise
- Dill
- Salt and pepper
- 1 Celery Stalk

Add
- 2 pieces of whole-wheat or gluten-free Toast
- Roma Tomato(Sliced)
- Small handful of Alfalfa Sprouts

(500 Calories)

Snack: 4-5 Medjool Dates
(250 calories)

Dinner: Stuffed Bell Peppers with Brown Rice, Vegan Cheese, Black Beans, and Onion
- 4 bell peppers
- 2/3 cup dry rice
- 1 cup vegan cheese
- 1 can black beans
- 1 onion
- Cilantro
- Salt

- Pepper
- Chili powder

(300 calories per pepper)

Dessert: Newman's Own Vegan Peanut Butter Cups (150 calories)

TOTAL CALORIES = 2050

The Basics of a Healthy Vegan Lifestyle

DAY 3 (5 Day Sample Meal Plan)

<u>Breakfast: Chocolate-Banana-Hemp Oatmeal</u>
- ½ cup oatmeal
- 2 bananas
- 1.5 tsp. cocoa powder
- 1 tbsp. hemp protein powder (or vegan protein powder of choice)
- Almond milk or water

Generally, I make the oatmeal first and then add the bananas. I like to put the banana slices on top of the oatmeal and warm them up for about 30 seconds to 1 minutes so I can mash them up in the oatmeal. It adds a sweetness to the bitterness of the cocoa
(400 Calories)

<u>Snack: Apple with Peanut Butter</u>
- 1 sliced apple
- 2 tbsp. peanut butter

(300 Calories)

<u>Lunch: Dahl (lentil Soup) and Pita Bread</u>
To make Dahl:
- 1 cup lentils of choice
- 3 cups water or vegetable stock

- 1 onion
- 2 potatoes
- 3 cloves garlic
- Turmeric
- Cumin
- Chili powder
- Bay leaves
- Ginger root
- Gram masala

First cook lentils in simmering stock, then combine all ingredients and let simmer

(makes 4 servings)

(200 Calories Lentils + 150 Pita) = 350 Calories

Snack:

Edamame (100 Calories)

2 peaches (100 calories)

Dinner: Vegan Spaghetti with Soy Meatballs
- Whole-grain or gluten free pasta
- Organic tomato sauce (or make your own!)
- One bag of soy meatballs

(Anywhere from 4-8 servings depending on portion size)

(400-600 Calories)

The Basics of a Healthy Vegan Lifestyle

<u>Dessert: Chocolate Covered Banana (Make your own, or try Diana's Frozen Bananas)</u>
(150 Calories)

TOTAL CALORIES: 1900

DAY 4 (5 Day Sample Meal Plan)

<u>Breakfast: Berry Chia Seed Pudding & Toast with Peanut Butter</u>

(Mix almond milk, chia seeds, and syrup in a jar and cover with lid. Place in fridge overnight)

- 1 cup almond milk
- 2 tsp. chia seeds
- 1 tbsp. maple syrup
- 1 cup fresh berries of your choice
- 2 pieces toast
- 1 -2 tbsp. peanut butter

(550 Calories Total)

<u>Snack: Crispy homemade Kale Chips & Carrots and Hummus</u>

(Put in oven at 300 for 20 minutes, check and flip)

- 1 bunch kale
- 1 tbsp. olive oil
- Salt and pepper

(250 Calories)

<u>Lunch: Spinach Smoothie Bowl</u>
- Heaping handful of spinach
- 2 scoops vegan protein powder
- 3 frozen bananas

The Basics of a Healthy Vegan Lifestyle

- ½ tbsp. maple syrup or agave to taste
- 1/3 cup water
- 1 cup frozen berries on top
- 1 tbsp. flax or chia seeds

(550 Calories)

Dinner: Roasted Sweet Potato, Beets, Asparagus, and Butternut Squash, with steamed Red cabbage and Brown Rice

- 1 medium-sized sweet potatoes
- 1-2 beets
- 10 asparagus spears
- 1 cup butternut squash
- 1 cup red cabbage
- 1 cup cooked brown rice

(Simple as it sounds to make, and oh so yummy! Season with nutritional yeast)

(550 Calories)

Dessert: Chocolate Banana Smoothie topped with coconut

- 1 tbsp. cocoa
- 2 frozen bananas
- 1 tbsp. agave syrup or maple syrup

- Shredded coconuts on top
(300 calories)

TOTAL CALORIES = 2200

The Basics of a Healthy Vegan Lifestyle

Day 5 (5 Day Sample Meal Plan)
Breakfast: Vegan Banana Split

- 1 banana
- 1 cup plain, unsweetened soy or coconut yogurt
- 1/2 granola of choice
- 1 cup blueberries
- 1 tbsp. maple or agave syrup if desired

(550 Calories)

Snack: Carrots and Bell Pepper with Hummus
(150 Calories)

Lunch: Portobello Mushroom Sandwich with Roasted Red Peppers and Pesto Sauce

(Broil Portobello mushroom in oven at 400-425 F for 20 minutes, turning over once. I coat mine with balsamic vinaigrette, salt and pepper)

- Portobello mushroom
- balsamic vinaigrette
- two pieces of toast
- pesto to spread on toast
- 4 roasted red peppers

(400 Calories)

Snack: Pear and Medjool Dates
(300 Calories)

Dinner: Black Bean Burritos with Guacamole, Vegan Cheese, Tomatoes, and Bell Pell Peppers

(To make homemade guacamole: smash up avocado, squeeze lemon juice over it and add salt and pepper-ta-da!)

This recipe can make 4 servings

- 1 can black beans
- 4 burritos
- 1 avocado
- Salt and pepper
- Lemon juice
- 1-2 cups vegan cheese
- 3 tomatoes
- 3 bell peppers

(550 Calories per burrito)

Dessert: Chocolate Covered Banana (150 Calories) – Diana's Bananas makes great ones, or you can make your own!)

TOTAL CALORIES: 2100

Lewis Haas

Chapter 6: One Size Never Fits All

One thing I cannot stress enough in a person's journey to veganism is that new followers need to make veganism work for them. True, you should abstain from all meat and dairy products but it is also okay to take one step at a time. If it is too much to abstain from honey or to stop wearing leather the first month you transition, then don't. If your favorite type of bread includes traces of egg, do not deprive yourself, at least not right away. It is better to ease into this lifestyle change so that it can last a lifetime. This chapter will talk about the non-dietary aspects of veganism that one can adapt to after growing accustomed to the vegan diet. Again, the choice to take up these habits is optional.

As noted, many vegans choose not to wear clothing made from animals such as wool (sheep), leather (cow), and even silk (worms) Vegans choose not to wear these textile sources because the process in which they are made often causes harm and pain to the animals, as described in previous chapters. Unless you are really compelled to, do not donate or throw away all your animal textiles at once. Rather, simply stop buying new leather shoes and silk scarves. Stop contributing to the textile economy by buying these items for yourself or for others. Stop giving others animal textiles as gifts. Finally, when you no longer feel the desire to wear these clothing items, then stop.

Some vegans prefer not to use cosmetic items and other various household items that used animal testing in the process of its development. This can be difficult to do because not all products are transparent about their use of animal testing. However, a 2013 ruling by the European Union (E.U.) made avoiding non-vegan items easier. The E.U. forbade the sale of all cosmetic products that used animal testing in their trials and developments.[45] This ban is not limited to the E.U. as it means companies worldwide that wish to sell their products in the EU must forgo animal testing.[46] Other countries like Israel followed suit. New vegans that do not live in the E.U. may choose to purchase vegan cosmetics and other products if they wish, but if it becomes daunting, they should cut themselves some slack. New

The Basics of a Healthy Vegan Lifestyle

vegans should purchase organic, vegan products but adhering to newfound veganism should never become a source of anxiety or distress. In essence, it is best if these things can be reasonably avoided, but that is not always possible and new vegans should not beat themselves up over it.

One vegan policy, for new and veteran vegans alike, is to remove honey from their diets. The way we currently produce honey in mass amounts is cruel and inhumane to bees. The fact is that bees feel pain, their colonies are split up, and they are forced to live in unnatural circumstances.[47] One of the most serious problems is that the world is facing a huge bee crisis. Bees are dying off in swarms (no pun intended) and they are necessary for the rest of the world's survival. Amazingly, one third of all plants need to be pollinated by bees. Using bees for honey production is selfish and wrong.[48]

You'll certainly have some mixed reactions from family members and friends about your transition and radically different lifestyle that includes no wool, honey or leather. What do you say to them? How do you respond? Should you start citing all the reasons they should be vegan, with statistics and PowerPoint slides to boot? Some vegans will choose to do this, and some will not. It doesn't necessarily mean that one vegan is truer to their lifestyle than another. It just means people choose to confront questions about their lifestyle differently.

At the very least, vegans should defend their beliefs and they should not eat animal products or give in to peer pressure. Nothing more is required of a vegan. However, if people respect a vegan's lifestyle or seem curious about, it would be great if a vegan were able to explain the reasoning behind their lifestyle and answer any questions. The more vegans in this world, the better! However, do not feel that you have to defend your beliefs to someone who is aggressive or rude. Unfortunately, these types of people are looking to start a fight. In essence, cite evidence as much or as little as you want when asked about your vegan lifestyle. Above all else, stay true to

The Basics of a Healthy Vegan Lifestyle

your convictions as a vegan and be proud of yourself for committing to this lifestyle.

Lewis Haas

Chapter 7: Eating Out

It is easy to stay to true to your vegan lifestyle in your own home, but eating out can be a challenge. Most restaurants use lard (animal fat-derived) in their cooking, or add cheese to any vegetarian dish. Angela Liddon, author of the magical vegan blog "Oh She Glows" came up with a wonderful guide to eating out at restaurants. I will share some of her tips that I have also found helpful in my quest to eat out as a vegan.

First, do your research. If you can pick a restaurant ahead of time and have a chance to look at its menu online you will be able to see whether or not vegan and vegetarian options are available. Angela mentions the website, "Happy Cow" to search for vegetarian and vegan options in your area. Likewise, you can use popular generic search engines like Yelp and Urban Spoon. Simply filter your results to show only vegan and vegetarian options. If menus are not available online, call the restaurant to ask what menu items they have for vegans.

Of course, planning ahead is not always an option and one must be improvise when, on a

Friday night, you suddenly find yourself with ten of your best meat-eating buddies. Like Angela, I suggest ethnic options. It's sad, but the standard American diet is one of the worst for one's health and for the environment. It is almost never vegan-friendly. Asian restaurants, especially Indian and Thai usually have vegan options. I have also found great luck at Middle Eastern restaurants. Falafel (baked or fried chickpea and flour balls) is almost always on the menu. Finally, Latin American restaurants often cater to vegetarians and vegans. Just ask them to hold the cheese in the fajitas. If these restaurants do not make the distinction between vegan and vegetarian options, request the waiter to make sure the chef cooks the food vegan. No oil from animals should be used. It also helps to tell them you have a lactose allergy as well to make sure they do not include dairy.

The worst-case scenario for a vegan may be trying to find something to eat at a BBQ, Irish Pub, or French restaurant. What do you do? In these cases, make a special request for select items. Ask for a modified version of one of their salads and a side or two (vegetables of the day, a side of rice, etc.). At the end of the day though, if

The Basics of a Healthy Vegan Lifestyle

you end up spending $20 on a house salad with nuts and a bowl of boiled vegetables, remember you are there for the company first, then the food. I like Angela's final tip most of all: "Don't sweat it."[49]

Lewis Haas

Chapter 8: Types of Vegans

Ambitious beginners to veganism may have heard of terms like Raw Vegan, 80/10/10, Raw till 4, High-Carb Low-Fat Vegan, or Plant-Based Vegan. I recommend transitioning to veganism first before trying these other types of veganism, but this chapter will shed some insight on to what these types of veganism are.

Raw Veganism, just as the name implies, is a vegan lifestyle that incorporates no cooked foods into the diet. At what temperature something is considered cooked varies, but it is safe to assume raw vegans are not going to be using an oven, microwave, or boiling water to cook any of their food. Thus, raw vegans eat produce-mainly fruits and soft vegetables. Raw vegans believe that when food is cooked at high temperatures some of the food's nutritional contents are destroyed. Though also believe eating food raw is the most natural and healthy state

Raw till 4 is a modified version of the raw vegan lifestyle. Raw till 4 followers eat raw food until their evening meal. Hence, the raw until 4 name. The raw till 4 diet, like the raw vegan diet, calls for followers to eat a minimum of 2500 or even 3000 calories a day in produce, especially fruit. Bananas tend to make up a large portion of this lifestyle.[50]

The 80/10/10 lifestyle comes from Dr. Douglas Graham. This diet program states that optimal health comes from a vegan a diet that is mainly raw - 80% carbohydrate, 10% protein, and 10% fat. The program also calls for monomeals, or meals in which you eat a large quantity of just one unprocessed item, like 10 bananas or 6 mangos.[51]

High-Carb Low-Fat Vegan (H.C.L.F.) lifestyle is very similar to these aforementioned lifestyles. This diet calls for no more than 10-15% of your calories come from fat. Many meals are raw and some may be monomeals, but this is not essential.

Finally, plant-based vegan is a name for a vegan who avoids any sort of processed food. They may or may not be H.C.L.F. vegan or raw vegans. Above all, they will not eat Oreos or Boca burgers since they are highly processed vegan products.

Conclusion

In addition to taking away clear and practical steps to transitioning to veganism, I hope readers have also learned that veganism is a flexible lifestyle change. Besides abstaining from the consumption of animal products, anything else goes. I wouldn't recommend it, but you could technically be a vegan who ate nothing but cinnamon toast crunch and soymilk. Veganism means something different to every vegan. It is an intensely personal lifestyle that often is not just restricted to a change in one's diet.

Vegans come in all shapes and sizes from all corners of the globe. One thing all vegans share, in all their wonderful diversity, is the compassionate call to eliminating the suffering of others. Something, some experience, or someone moved you to consider veganism. Often, it is a combination of the three. When the going is tough and when roadblocks are in your way, take a deep breath and remind yourself of this call and your noble cause. You have the call, the will, and the drive. This book is here to help you along your path.

Thank You

Thank you for downloading my book and I hope you enjoyed it and found many things insightful. Furthermore, you can opt-in to my Book Notification Group to get all the latest information on free promotions, discounts and future book releases. Go to http://eepurl.com/bfE46z to get signed up.

I would really appreciate if you would take a minute to post a review on Amazon about this book. I check all my reviews and love to get feedback (this is the real reward for me - knowing that I'm helping others).

If you have any friends or family that may enjoy this book, please spread the love and gift it to them.

View my other work at Amazon Author Central.

About the Author

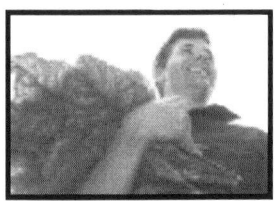

Lewis Haas is a father of 3 girls and a freelance writer. He enjoys daily meditation, exercising and spending time with his family. Currently residing in Tampa, Florida, his favorite time of year is winter when he meditates in the great outdoors.

References

About the FoodnSport Team. (n.d). FoodnSport: Defining the Cause of Health Retrieved from http://foodnsport.com/about/

Ask the Experts: Dairy Products. (n.d.) Physicians Committee for Responsible Medicine. Retrieved from http://pcrm.org/health/cancer-resources/ask/ask-the-expert-dairy- products

Being a Vegetarian. (n.d.). Retrieved from Brown University Health Promotion website: http://www.brown.edu/Student_Services/Health_Services/Health_Education/nutrition_&_eating_concerns/being_a_vegetarian.php

Definition of Veganism. (n.d.). The Vegan Society. Retrieved from: https://www.vegansociety.com/try-vegan/definition-veganism

Campbell, C. T. & Campbell, T. M. (2006). *The China Study: Startling Implications for Diet,*

References

Weight Loss and Long-Term Health. Dallas, TX: BenBella Books

Casalena, Nina. (2011, December 5). The Vegetarian Resource Group Blog: How Many Adults are Vegan in the U.S.?. Retrieved from: http://www.vrg.org/blog/2011/12/05/how-many-adults-are-vegan-in-the-u-s/

Compassion for Animals. (n.d.). The Vegan Society. Retrieved from http://www.vegansociety.com/sites/default/files/CompassionForAnimalsedited.pdf

Cosmetics and Household-Product Animal Testing. (n.d.) People for the Ethical Treatment of Animals (PETA). Retrieved from http://www.peta.org/issues/animals-used-for-experimentation/cosmetic-household-products-animal-testing/

Craig, Winston J. (2009). Health Effects of Vegan Diets. *The American Journal of Clinical Nutrition.* Available from: http://ajcn.nutrition.org/content/89/5/1627S.full

Davis, John. (2010-2012). *World Veganism – Past, Present, and Future.* Retrieved from: http://www.ivu.org/history/Vegan_History.pdf

References

Fish And Other Sea Animals Used For Food. (n.d.) People for the Ethical Treatment Animals. Retrieved from
http://www.peta.org/issues/animals-used-for-food/factory-farming/fish/

Food, Farm Animals, and Drugs. (n.d.) Natural Resources Defense Council. Retrieved from http://www.nrdc.org/food/saving-antibiotics.asp

From Shell to Hell: The Modern Egg Industry. (2015). Animal Aid. Retrieved from http://www.animalaid.org.uk/h/n/CAMPAIGNS/factory/ALL/578/

Graham, Douglass. (2006). *The 80/10/10 Diet.* Key Largo, FL: FoodnSport Press

Grossman, Elizabeth. (2013, April 30). Declining Bee Populations Pose A Threat to Global Agriculture. *Yale: Environment 360* [Blog Post] Retrieved from
http://e360.yale.edu/feature/declining_bee_populations_pose_a_threat_to_global agriculture/2645/

Healthy Diet. (May 2015). The World Health Organization. Retrieved from http://www.who.int/mediacentre/factsheets/fs394/en/

References

History. (n.d.) The Vegan Society. Retrieved from https://www.vegansociety.com/society/history

Hyman, Mark. (2010, July 10). Dairy: 6 Reasons You Should Avoid It At All Costs or Why Following the USDA Food Pyramid Guidelines is Bad for Your Health. *The Huffington Post.* Retrieved from http://www.huffingtonpost.com/dr-mark-hyman/dairy-free-dairy-6-reason_b_558876.html

Kotz, Deborah. (2008, June 23). Time in the Sun: How Much is Needed for Vitamin D? *U.S. News & World Report: Health.* Retrieved from http://health.usnews.com/health-news/family-health/heart/articles/2008/06/23/time-in-the-sun-how-much-is-needed-for-vitamin-d

Lambert, C. P., Frank, L. L. & Evans, W. J. (2004). Macronutrient Considerations for the Sport of Bodybuilding. *Sports Medicine, 34.* 317-327.

Lewis, Noah. (n.d.). Why Honey Is Not Vegan. Retrieved from http://vegetus.org/honey/honey.htm

References

Liddon, Angela. (2013, June 2). 10 Tips for Eating Out as Vegan [Blog Post Retrieved from http://libguides.gwumc.edu/c.php?g=27779&p=1 70343

Lohan, Tara. (2010, January 25). Got Milk? A Disturbing Look at the Dairy Industry. *Alternet.* Retrieved from http://www.alternet.org/story/145378/got_milk_a_disturbing_look_at_the_dairy_in dustry

More Reasons to Go Vegan. (n.d.). People for the Ethical Treatment of Animals. Retrieved from http://www.peta.org/issues/animals-used-for-food/reasons-go-   vegan/

Nelson, K. J., & Zeratsky, K. (2011, February 22). Nutrion-Wise Blog: Should You Be a Flexitarian? [Mayo Clinic Official Blog] Retrieved from http://www.mayoclinic.org/healthy-lifestyle/nutrition-and-healthy-eating/expert-blog/flexitarian/bgp-20056276

Pau, Jackie. (2010, May 13). The Dirty Dozen and Clean 15 of Produce. [Blog Post] Need to Know on PBS. Retrieved from http://www.pbs.org/wnet/need-to-

References

know/health/the-dirty-dozen-and-clean-15-of-produce/616/

Pesctarian. [Def. 1]. (2015). *Oxford Dictionary.* Retrieved May 18, 2011, from http://www.oxforddictionaries.com/us/definition/american_english/pescatarian

Podell, Reina. (2014, March 11). How the Dairy Lobby Convinced Americans that Cow's Milk = The Best Source of Calcium. *One Green Planet.* Retrieved from http://www.onegreenplanet.org/vegan-food/dairy-lobby-cows-milk-calcium/

Protein. (2012, October 4). The Centers for Disease Control and Prevention. Retrieved from http://www.cdc.gov/nutrition/everyone/basics/protein.html#How%20much%20protein

Raw Till 4 Diet Plan Menus. (n.d.) My Raw Till 4 Life [Blog] Retrieved from http://rawtill4diet.com/raw-till-4-diet-plan

Spotlight: Livestock Impacts on the Environment. (2016, November). Food and Agriculture Organization of the United Nations. Retrieved from http://www.fao.org/ag/magazine/0612sp1.htm

References

Truath, Erin. (2014, January 16). *Is 2014 the Year of the Vegan?* [Web log comment]. Retrieved from http://www.onegreenplanet.org/news/is-2014-the-year-of-the- vegan/

Walsh, Bryan. (2013, December 13). The Triple Whooper Environmental Impact of Global Meat Production. *Times Magazine.* Retrieved from http://science.time.com/2013/12/16/the-triple-whopper-environmental-impact-of-global-meat-production/

What Is a Factory Farm? (2015). American Society for the Prevention of Cruelty to Animals. Retrieved from https://www.aspca.org/fight-cruelty/farm-animal- cruelty/what-factory-farm

The Wool Industry. (n.d.). People for the Ethical Treatment of Animals (PETA). Retrieved from http://www.peta.org/issues/animals-used-for-clothing/wool- industry/

Vitamin B12. (2011, June 24). National Institutes of Health: Office of Dietary Supplements. Retrieved from http://ods.od.nih.gov/factsheets/VitaminB12-HealthProfessional/#h3

References

Vitamin D. (2014, November 4). National Institutes of Health: Office of Dietary Supplements. Retrieved from: http://ods.od.nih.gov/factsheets/VitaminD-HealthProfessional/#h3

References

Citations

[1] Nelson & Zeratsky, 2011.
[2] "Pescatarian," 2015.
[3] Casalena, 2011.
[4] "Being a Vegetarian," n.d..
[5] "Definition of Veganism," 2015.
[6] Lohan, 2010.
[7] ibid
[8] ibid
[9] "From Shell to Hell: The Modern Egg Industry," 2015.
[10] ibid
[11] Hyman, 2010 July 1.
[12] "Ask the Expert: Dairy Products," n.d.
[13] "About the FoodnSport Team," n.d.
[14] Graham, 2006, p. 28.
[15] "History," n.d.
[16] ibid.
[17] Trauth, 2014 January 16.
[18] Campbell & Campbell, 2006.
[19] Craig does criticize some potential nutritional deficiencies in the Vegan diet, including Vitamin D, Calcium, and B-12. These are common misconceptions that will be explained in a later chapter of this book.
[20] "More Reasons to Go Vegan," n.d.
[21] "What is a Factory Farm?" n.d.
[22] "Compassion for Animals," n.d.
[23] "Fish and Other Sea Animals Used for Food," n.d.

References

[24] ibid
[25] "The Wool Industry," n.d.
[26] Walsh, 2013 December 16.
[27] ibid
[28] "Spotlight: Livestock Impacts on the Environment," November 2006
[29] "Food, Farm Animals, and Drugs" n.d.
[30] "Healthy Diet," May 2014.
[31] ibid
[32] "Protein" 2012, October 4.
[33] Lambert, C. P., Frank, L. L., & Evans, W. J., 2004, 318.
[34] Campbell, 37.
[35] Campbell, 31-32
[36] "Vitamin B12," 2011, June 24.
[37] ibid
[38] Graham, 254.
[39] People living in northern climates will not be able to get their Vitamin D from the sun during the winter months. In the United States and the Eastern seaboard this is anywhere north of Atlanta
[40] Kotz, 2008.
[41] Podell, 2014 March 11.
[42] Campbell, 178, 199-201, 208-210
[43] (Pau, 2010, May 13).
[44] ibid
[45] "Cosmetic and Household Product Animal Testing," n.d.
[46] ibid
[47] Lewis, n.d.).

References

[48] Grossman, 2013, April 30.
[49] Liddon, 2013
[50] "Raw till 4 Diet Plan Menus," n.d.
[51] Graham, 259.

Printed in Great Britain
by Amazon